Time to try.....

KETO

GREEN

SMOOTHIES

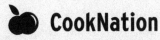 CookNation

Time to try... Ketogenic Green Smoothies

Delicious Keto smoothies for weight loss, detox & cleanse

ISBN 978-1-912511-51-8

DISCLAIMER

The content of this book is also available under the title 'Ketogenic Green Smoothies' by CookNation. Except for use in any review, the reproduction or utilisation of this work in whole or in part in any form by any electronic, mechanical or other means, now known or hereafter invented, including xerography, photocopying and recording, or in any information storage or retrieval system, is forbidden without the permission of the publisher.
This book is sold subject to the condition that it shall not, by way of trade or otherwise, be lent, resold, hired out or otherwise circulated without the prior consent of the publisher in any form of binding or cover other than that in which it is published and without a similar condition including this condition being imposed on the subsequent purchaser.
This book is designed to provide information on the popular Ketogenic Diet. Some recipes may contain nuts or traces of nuts. Those suffering from any allergies associated with nuts should avoid any recipes containing nuts or nut based oils.

This information is provided and sold with the knowledge that the publisher and author do not offer any legal or other professional advice.
In the case of a need for any such expertise consult with the appropriate professional.
This book does not contain all information available on the subject, and other sources of recipes are available.
Every effort has been made to make this book as accurate as possible. However, there may be typographical and or content errors. Therefore, this book should serve only as a general guide and not as the ultimate source of subject information.
This book contains information that might be dated and is intended only to educate and entertain.
The author and publisher shall have no liability or responsibility to any person or entity regarding any loss or damage incurred, or alleged to have incurred, directly or indirectly, by the information contained in this book.

CONTENTS

Energising Green Smoothies   45

Full Keto Smoothies 83

INTRODUCTION

The keto diet is well known for its great ability to turn the body into a fat burning machine.

For those looking to lose weight and improve their overall health, the Ketogenic diet is a great tool to turn to. As with any diet or eating plan though, it is essential to be a little organised, so you are able to stick to eating the correct foods and to stay focused. Making sure you are still consuming a wealth of vitamins and minerals and avoiding carbohydrates can be a challenge, which is where we can help.

Our collection of delicious smoothies & juices have been designed to complement your existing Keto diet. Most are green but we've sneaked in a few mixed smoothies too to add some variety. Some of our smoothies can be used as a meal replacement, if your goal is weight loss and therefore each is calorie counted, however we suggest our smoothies are best used as part of your overall Keto eating plan.

Devised to detox your body we suggest you consume 2-3 smoothies from the detox and energising chapters of this book for 10 consecutive days as part of your balanced daily Keto diet. This will help rid your body of unwanted and harmful toxins and leave you feeling energised and cleansed whilst setting you on a path to sustained weight loss. The final chapter 'Full Keto' will keep you inspired long term. You should introduce smoothies from this chapter after your initial 10 day detox period.

But what is Keto?

There are numerous types of Keto eating plans out there, but Ketogenic Green Smoothies follows basic, standard principles; working on the belief that the body benefits from eating easy to digest and unprocessed foods is important, plus consuming minimal carbohydrate and high levels of animal-based proteins, natural plant fats, vegetables, nuts and seeds is the core of a Keto diet.

Essentially this method is aimed to programme the body to use its unwanted stores of fat, instead of burning the sugary carbohydrates that are more usually consumed. By restricting these carbohydrates, you begin to re-programme your body to use the fat stores, instead of the glycogen stores in the muscles – this process is known as ketosis.

Once you have hit 'full' Ketosis and your body is in this high gear, you will find your metabolism is increased and the quality of the Keto food you consume will provide you with lots of energy and more mental alertness. Afternoon "slumps" are less likely to be experienced due to the fact you are eating adequate nutrition. Ordinarily reducing calories to achieve weight loss can result in low moods and agitation however this too can be avoided when eating a Keto diet as you will be reducing carbohydrates but not reducing calories and nutrition!

How Do You Know You're in Full Ketosis?

When your body is functioning at this level it is breaking down Ketones (fats and fatty acids) for energy, rather than the glucose from carbohydrates. As a result you should experience the following:

- Excess weight loss
- Loss of appetite
- Increased focus and energy
- Less energy dips
- Increased urination

The potential Benefits?

The Ketogenic Diet brings many benefits to your health and long term, it can really help with chronic health issues.

- Reduction in weight
- Lowered insulin levels and reduced risk of developing Type II Diabetes
- Clearer skin
- Better control of epilepsy
- Increased levels of good cholesterol
- Lower blood pressure
- Reduced risk of developing brain disease.

What to Eat?

Protein such as beef, lamb, pork, chicken, venison, fish, seafood & tofu. Try to use grass fed, organic and sustainably sourced where possible.

Eggs: Organic

Dairy Products: full fat and organic, real butter, cream and cheeses. Always avoid low fat, sugary varieties.

Vegetables: asparagus, spinach, all types of cabbage, mushrooms, peppers, tomatoes, cucumber, olives, courgette, aubergine, etc.

Nuts and Seeds: almonds, macadamia, brazil nuts, hazelnuts, walnuts, pumpkin seeds, chia seeds, sesame seeds, sunflower seeds, etc.

Fruits: raspberries, blueberries, strawberries and blackberries (only in moderation though and exclude if you are on a weight loss goal).

Natural Fats: avocado oil, sesame oil, olive oil and coconut oil.

Drinks: coconut water, tea and coffee, with cream.

Foods to avoid include: starchy root vegetables; processed food; sugary food; energy drinks; grains & beans.

Ketogenic Green Smoothies make life easy by helping keep you inspired with a broad spectrum of vital plant compounds and animal-based proteins to complement your overall keto eating plan.

Notes On Blenders

There are many high-speed blenders out there on the market of various designs. Many have an upside-down cup and described as a "bullet" and some come with extra cups and drinks tops. They take up minimal space in the cupboard or on a work surface, for quick access.   This makes creating smoothies and healthy drinks so easy to work into a busy schedule.

Many vegetable smoothies and juices taste even better iced cold. These blender "bullets" are great at smashing through ice cubes to add to your drink, to create some lovely crushed ice concoctions.

It's worth investing in a good quality appliance. When you use a kitchen appliance daily, it's usually worth every penny spent! However, all of these recipes can still be made in a food processor of most designs, so there is no need to purchase expensive gadgets when getting started. Use the smallest bowl ones and soak the nuts or seeds overnight if possible, to help make processing the ingredients a little less work.

Tips On Blending

To make the most of your blending, follow these tips:

- Always use the freshest ingredients possible.
- Chop ingredients, especially harder produce, into small pieces to ensure
- smoother blending.
- Wash vegetables and fruit really well before use.
- Once a smoothie or drink has been processed, it will begin to lose its nutritional value, so it is best to consume as soon as possible after being made.
- If you want to prepare ahead, add everything to the blender cup and store in the fridge until the last minute and then blend just before needed.
- You can use a variety of frozen fruits and vegetables for these recipes. It will make the drinks icy cold and sometimes quite "slushie" which is great for a hot day or for after a hard work out!
- You can freeze avocados to be used for smoothies (their texture after freezing is not suitable for slicing on to a dish). You can remove the stone, peel and then mash half an avocado with a little lemon juice. Store these individually in little freezer bags so you can remove as and when you need for single portions.
- Adding ½ tsp of coconut oil to smoothies and drinks can be a welcome addition if you wish to increase the fat content a little in your Keto diet. When stored at a reasonably warm room temperature, the oil will almost be a liquid so easy to reach for and spoon out.
- If you find you can't get all of the ingredients into your blender in one go, add some of them and then blend to make room. Add the rest and continue.
- Make sure the blender is unplugged before disassembling or cleaning.
- Set aside the power base and blade holders as these should not be used in a dishwasher.
- Use hot soapy water to clean the blades but do not immerse in boiling water as this can warp the plastic.
- Use a damp cloth to clean the power base.
- All cups and lids can be placed in a dishwasher.
- For stubborn marks inside the cup, fill the cup 2/3 full of warm soapy water and screw on the milling blade. Attached to the power base and run for 20-30 seconds.
- During cleaning or use do not put your hands or any utensils near the moving blade. Always ensure the blender/food processor is unplugged when assembling/disassembling or cleaning.

The type of blender you have will dictate which seeds and skins should be removed from fruit and vegetables. However the following seeds and pits should always be removed before blending as they may contain chemicals which can release cyanide into the body when ingested so do not use any of the following in your smoothies:

* Apple Seeds   * Cherry Pits   *Peach pits   * Apricot Pits   * Plum Pits

The different drinks and smoothies in Ketogenic Green Smoothies are split into three categories: Detox, Energising and Full Keto which give you a choice of recipes depending on your mood or requirements.

Detox

This section gives you a number of drink recipes using water or coconut water as a base. Coconut water is a natural, hydrating drink which provides calcium, phosphorus, magnesium, sodium and potassium. It is the drink of choice for many athletes and is a great choice to blend with foods to produce nutritious drinks.

Allowing the body to rest from working hard to remove toxins from our body, is essential for our health. This can be done by eliminating as many toxic foods from your diet as possible and also by consuming the vegetables and herbs that will assist your body with the detoxification process. Cleansing and hydrating drinks with natural ingredients from many different sources is a great addition to a Keto diet.

Energising

This section has a wealth of recipes to inspire you to keep to your dietary objectives. When faced with inadequate nutrition, it is easy to reach for foods that are restricted just because it is easy. These energising drinks will provide you with energy and proteins, needed for repair and growth, so you remain positive and full of vitality.

Many of these drinks use unsweetened almond milk, coconut milk, nuts, seeds and nut butters as a base and provide the essential good fats needed on a Keto diet. They will keep you feeling fuller for longer and some of these could be used as meal replacements if you are trying to lose weight. Give some of these flavour combinations a go, as you may be surprised.

Full Keto

These drinks are aimed towards those who have settled into a great Keto eating plan and have embraced the changes. Using ingredients that are typically high in animal proteins and fats and some ingredients that should only be eaten in moderation, these drinks provide some well-loved flavours. Life is short and whatever eating plan you follow, everyone loves a treat from time to time (note: if you are on a weight loss programme, you may only want to dip into these recipes occasionally).

Many of these drinks use single cream, but this can be substituted with whipping cream or even cream cheese and sour cream. Try to aim for dairy creams that are 40% fat and higher for the best results.

Ketogenic Green Smoothies is inspiration and motivation to keep adequately hydrated and nourished whilst eating a Keto diet. Yes, there are a number of foods that need to be avoided, but you can celebrate and enjoy the foods you CAN eat. Try out some of these great flavour combinations knowing they have been designed to taste great and to give your wellbeing a well-deserved boost.

About CookNation

CookNation is the leading publisher of innovative and practical recipe books for the modern, health conscious cook.

CookNation titles bring together delicious, easy and practical recipes with their unique no-nonsense approach - making cooking for diets and healthy eating fast, simple and fun. With a range of #1 best-selling titles - from the innovative 'Skinny' calorie-counted series, to the 5:2 Diet Recipes collection - CookNation recipe books prove that 'Diet' can still mean 'Delicious'!

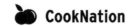 CookNation

Time to try....

KETO

GREEN

SMOOTHIES

Detox

DETOX KALE & CELERY

190 calories

······· *Ingredients* ·······

CLEANSING

- 225g/8oz kale
- 1 stalk off celery
- 250ml/8½floz coconut water
- Avocado
- 1 tbsp fresh flat leaf parsley
- Water

······· *Method* ·······

1 Rinse the kale and remove any thick stalks.

2 Rinse the celery well.

3 Add all of the ingredients into a high speed blender.

4 Add a little water if needed to make up to the level that will fill your smoothie glass.

5 Blend the ingredients together until really smooth. Enjoy immediately.

CHEF'S NOTE
Celery is believed to cleanse the blood.

WARM SPICE CLEANSE

155 calories

Ingredients

- 75g/3oz kale
- 250ml/8½floz coconut water
- 150g/5oz yellow or orange bell pepper
- Pinch of cumin
- ½ tbsp fresh grated ginger
- ½ tsp turmeric (fresh or ground)
- Water

Method

1 Rinse the kale and remove any thick stalks

2 Rinse the bell pepper and remove any seeds. Roughly chop.

3 Add all the ingredients to a high-speed blender and top up with enough water if needed, to make up to the level to fill your smoothie glass.

4 Process the ingredients until really smooth. Enjoy immediately.

CHEF'S NOTE
Peppers are packed with anti-oxidants.

GARDENER'S CLEANSE

259 calories

Ingredients

- 50g/2oz baby beetroot leaves
- 50g/2oz baby spinach leaves
- 250ml/8½floz coconut water
- 1 tbsp fresh flat leaf parsley
- 75g/3oz courgette
- 50g/2oz whole almonds
- Water

Method

1 Rinse the baby leaves well and drain.

2 Rinse the courgette and roughly chop. Leave the skin and seeds intact.

3 Add everything to a high-speed blender.

4 Top with a little water if need be, so the level will fill your smoothie glass.

5 Blend the ingredients really well until smooth. Enjoy immediately.

CHEF'S NOTE
Parsley is associated with helping the kidneys and liver to detox.

FRESH GREEN CLEANSE

230 calories

Ingredients

- 2 celery stalks
- 300g/11oz cucumber
- 125g/4oz kale
- 225g/8oz spinach
- 1 tbsp fresh coriander
- 1 lemon
- 1 lime
- Water

Method

1 Wash the celery, spinach, cucumber, coriander and drain.

2 Cut any thick green stalks off the kale and rinse well.

3 Peel and de-seed the lemon and lime.

4 Add all of the ingredients to a high-speed blender and add enough water to a level that will fill your smoothie glass.

5 Process the ingredients until smooth. Enjoy immediately.

CHEF'S NOTE
Coriander is known to support liver function and is a great detox ingredient.

SUPER GREEN SLUSH

116 calories

Ingredients

VITAMINS C & K

- 125g/4oz cucumber
- 50g/2oz baby spinach leaves
- 1 tbsp fresh mint leaves
- 250ml/8½floz coconut water
- 1 tbsp lemon juice
- 2 handfuls of ice

Method

1 Rinse the spinach and drain well.

2 Rinse the cucumber and roughly chop but leave the skin and seeds intact.

3 Rinse the mint leaves.

4 Add all of the ingredients into a high-speed blender.

5 Process the ingredients until quite smooth but still icy and fresh.

6 Enjoy immediately

CHEF'S NOTE
Mint is a great in a detox drink, it's fresh tasting and full of soothing properties.

DETOX ITALIAN

123 calories

Ingredients

PROTEIN RICH

- 100g/3½oz aubergine
- 4 black olives
- 250ml/8 ½floz coconut water
- 1 tsp rosemary leaves
- 1 small garlic clove
- Water

Method

1 Rinse and roughly chop the aubergine

2 Crush the garlic clove.

3 Add all of the ingredients into a high-speed blender and add enough water to a level that will fill your smoothie glass.

4 Process the ingredients until smooth. This may take a little longer to ensure the rosemary is broken down. Enjoy immediately.

CHEF'S NOTE

Rosemary is known to both help the liver detox and to improve brain function.

YELLOW GINGER CLEANSE

128 calories

.... *Ingredients* ....

- 2cm/1 inch fresh root ginger
- 150g/5oz kale
- 125g/4oz broccoli

- 250ml/8½floz coconut water
- ½ tsp turmeric
- Water

.... *Method* ....

1 Prepare the ginger and grate into the cup of a high speed blender.

2 Rinse the broccoli and cut into small pieces.

3 Add all of the ingredients into the blender and top up with enough water to a level that will fill your smoothie glass.

4 Blend until the ingredients are really smooth.

5 Enjoy immediately.

CHEF'S NOTE
The turmeric adds a lovely yellow hue to this drink and has anti-inflammatory benefits.

BAMBOO HYDRATOR

120
calories

Ingredients

- 175g/6oz bamboo shoots
- 200g/7 oz bok choi
- 125g/4oz cucumber

- 250ml/8½floz coconut water
- 3-4 fennel seeds
- Water

Method

1 Drain and rinse the bamboo shoots (if using canned)

2 Rinse the bok choi and roughly chop.

3 Rinse the cucumber and roughly chop, leaving the skin and seeds intact,

4 Add all the ingredients into a high-speed blender and top up with enough water to reach a level that will fill your smoothie glass.

5 Process the ingredients until really smooth. Enjoy immediately.

CHEF'S NOTE
Bamboo shoots are a great source of fibre that is sometimes hard to find on a keto diet.

VITAMIN C BOOSTER

193 calories

Ingredients

HELPS FIGHT ILLNESS

- 175g/6oz red bell pepper
- 125g/4 oz kale
- 200ml/7floz coconut water
- 1 tsp grated ginger root
- ½ tsp turmeric
- Water

Method

1 Rinse the bell pepper and roughly chop, removing the seeds.

2 Rinse the kale and remove any thick stems.

3 Prepare the ginger root and grate in to a blender.

4 Add all of the other ingredients in to the blender and top up with enough water so the level will fill you glass.

5 Process the ingredients until really smooth. Enjoy immediately.

CHEF'S NOTE
Red bell peppers and kale together provide wonderful sources of vitamin C, essential to see you through cold season.

BABY LEAF HYDRATOR

94 calories

Ingredients

BONE BUILDER →

- 75g/3oz baby beetroot leaves
- 75g/3oz baby spinach leaves
- 250ml/8½floz coconut water
- 1 tbsp flat leaf parsley leaves
- 3-4 whole almonds
- Water

Method

1 Rinse the baby leaves and parsley, drain well.,

2 Roughly chop the almonds to help the processing a little.

3 Add all of the ingredients into a high-speed blender and top with enough water to bring to a level to fill your glass.

4 Process the ingredients until really smooth. Enjoy immediately.

CHEF'S NOTE

The baby leaves used in this drink will help improve calcium levels.

MINT AND WATERCRESS DETOX

90 calories

Ingredients

FIGHTS ILLNESS

- 150g/5oz watercress leaves
- 1 tbsp mint leaves
- 250ml/8½floz coconut water
- 75g/3oz asparagus spears
- Water

Method

1 Rinse the watercress and mint well, Drain.

2 Clean the asparagus and roughly chop, removing any really fibrous stem.

3 Place the ingredients into a high-speed blender and top up with enough water to enable you to fill your glass.

4 Blend the ingredients until really smooth.

5 Enjoy immediately.

CHEF'S NOTE

Watercress provides a great source of vitamin C and can help fight illness.

THE GREEN MACHINE

136 calories

Ingredients

- 125g/4oz cucumber
- 1 celery stalk
- 150g/5oz kale
- 250ml/8½floz coconut water
- 1 tbsp lemon juice
- 1 tbsp lime juice
- 1 tbsp coriander leaves
- Water

Method

1 Rinse the cucumber and roughly chop, leaving the seeds and skin intact.

2 Rinse the kale and remove any thick stems.

3 Rinse and drain the coriander leaves.

4 Add all of the ingredients into a high-speed blender and top up with enough water to fill the glass you are using,

5 Blend the ingredients really well and until smooth. Enjoy immediately.

CHEF'S NOTE
The added coriander can also help ease indigestion and bloating.

BROCCOLI SALAD DETOX

145 calories

Ingredients

- 150g/5oz broccoli
- 150g/5oz romaine lettuce leaves
- 75g/3oz baby spinach leaves
- 1 tbsp oregano

- 250ml/8½floz coconut water
- Water

Method

1 Rinse and roughly chop the broccoli florets.

2 Rinse and drain the romaine, spinach and oregano leaves

3 Add all of the ingredients into a high-speed blender and top up with enough extra water to fill a smoothie glass.

4 Process the ingredients until well blended. Enjoy immediately.

CHEF'S NOTE

Broccoli is a vegetable that really benefits the blood. It provides Vitamin K, which improves blood clotting.

RED RADISH DETOX

108 calories

Ingredients

VITAMIN E BOOST

- 200g/7oz red radishes
- 150g/5oz white cabbage
- 1 tbsp thyme leaves
- 250ml/8½floz coconut water
- Water

Method

1 Rinse the radishes and remove the green stalks on each.

2 Rinse and core the cabbage and roughly chop.

3 Rinse and drain the thyme.

4 Add everything to a high-speed blender and add enough water to fill the glass you are using.

5 Process all of the ingredients until smooth.

6 Enjoy immediately.

CHEF'S NOTE
Vitamin E is an essential nutrient to balance hormones.

GARLIC CLEANSER

Ingredients

- 200g/7oz cauliflower
- 1 garlic clove
- 50g courgette
- 1 tsp lemon juice

- 250ml/8½floz coconut water
- 1 tbsp parsley
- Water

Method

1 Rinse the cauliflower well and roughly chop.

2 Rinse the courgette and roughly chop, leaving the skin and seeds intact.

3 Wash the parsley leaves and drain well.

4 Add all of the ingredients into a high speed blender and top up with water to make enough liquid to fill your glass.

5 Blend the ingredients together until smooth. Enjoy immediately.

CHEF'S NOTE
Garlic is known for its great anti-oxidant abilities, maybe chew some mint leaves after though!

ALFALFA HERBAL DETOX

89 calories

Ingredients

ANTI-AGING →

- 75g/3oz alfalfa sprouts
- 2 stalks of celery
- 1 tsp sage leaves
- 1 tsp thyme
- 1 tbsp lemon juice
- 250ml/8½floz coconut water
- Water

Method

1 Rinse the alfalfa really well and drain.

2 Rinse the celery stalks and roughly chop.

3 Rinse the herbs and drain.

4 Add everything to a high-speed blender and top up with water so there is enough liquid to fill your glass.

5 Blend until really smooth. Enjoy immediately.

CHEF'S NOTE

It is thought that alfalfa sprouts have great anti-ageing and anti-oxidant benefits.

ASPARAGUS REFRESHER

110 calories

Ingredients

ANTIOXIDANT +

- 150g/5oz asparagus
- 125g/4oz cucumber
- 250ml/8½floz coconut water
- 1 lemon
- 1 tbsp flat leaf parsley leaves
- Ice cubes

Method

1 Wash and roughly chop the asparagus, removing any fibrous stems at the end.

2 Wash and roughly chop the cucumber, leaving skin and seeds intact.

3 Wash and peel the lemon.

4 Wash and drain the parsley.

5 Add all of the ingredients into a high-speed blender.

6 When smooth, add handfuls of ice and process again, to create a hydrating, slushie drink.

CHEF'S NOTE
Asparagus can help detoxify the liver and kidneys and has a generally cleansing effect on your body's other systems.

HERBAL DETOX JUICE

142 calories

Ingredients

- 50g/2oz kale
- 150g/5oz courgette
- 1 stalk of celery
- 1 tbsp flat leaf parsley
- 1 tbsp oregano leaves

- 5 black olives, pitted
- 200ml/7floz coconut water
- 1 tbsp lemon juice
- Water

Method

1 Rinse the kale and celery.

2 Cut the thick stems from the kale and roughly chop.

3 Rinse and roughly chop the courgette, leaving the skin and seeds intact.

4 Rinse the parsley and oregano, drain.

5 Add all of the ingredients into a high-speed blender and add a little water if need be.

6 Process until the ingredients are smooth. Enjoy immediately.

CHEF'S NOTE
Oregano and parsley are both diuretics that help flush toxins from your body.

TOMATO DETOX

126 calories

Ingredients

LYCOPENE →

- 150g plum tomatoes
- 250ml/8½ coconut water
- 100g/3½oz aubergine
- 1 garlic clove
- 1 tbsp basil leaves
- Water and ice

Method

1 Rinse the tomatoes and roughly chop.

2 Rinse the aubergine and roughly chop.

3 Crush the garlic clove and add it to a high-speed blender.

4 Rinse the basil and drain.

5 Add all of the ingredients to the blender and top up with water if need be, so the level fills the glass you are using.

6 Blend the ingredients until smooth. This smoothie is particularly nice with lots of crushed ice. Enjoy immediately.

CHEF'S NOTE
Tomatoes are a great source of lycopene, a useful anti-oxidant which aids detox.

SAUERKRAUT & DILL CLEANSE

143 calories

Ingredients

- 60g/2½oz sauerkraut
- 100g/3½oz cauliflower
- 250ml/8½floz coconut water
- 1 lemon
- 1 tbsp fresh dill
- water

Method

1 Drain the sauerkraut well.

2 Rinse the cauliflower and roughly chop in to small florets.

3 Wash the dill and drain,

4 Peel and roughly chop the lemon.

5 Add all of the ingredients into a high-speed blender, topping up with water if necessary so you can fill your glass.

6 Process the ingredients until smooth. Enjoy immediately,

CHEF'S NOTE
Sauerkraut is full of beta-carotene which works as a great anti-oxidant. It is known to improve gut bacteria and helpful during a detox.

SPROUT TOP SMOOTHIE

185 calories

Ingredients

- 125g/4 Brussels sprout tops
- 125g/4oz cauliflower
- 125g/4oz cucumber
- 1 tbsp coriander leaves

- 250ml/8½floz coconut water
- 1 tbsp lemon juice
- Water

Method

1 Rinse the Brussels sprout tops and drain. Roughly chop.

2 Wash and roughly chop the cauliflower.

3 Rinse the cucumber and roughly chop, leaving the skin and seeds intact.

4 Add all of the ingredients to a high-speed blender and add a little more water, to reach the level that will fill your glass.

5 Blend until all of the ingredients are smooth. Enjoy immediately,

CHEF'S NOTE
Brussels sprout tops aren't widely used but are a cheap way to pack your diet with Vitamin C, perfect for a detox programme.

LEMON VERBENA & CUCUMBER CLEANSER

118 calories

Ingredients

SUPER HYDRATOR

- 3 tbsp lemon verbena leaves
- 150g/5oz cucumber
- 2 stalks of celery
- 250ml/8½floz coconut water
- 1 tsp mint leaves
- Water and ice

Method

1 Rinse and drain the lemon verbena and mint leaves.

2 Wash and roughly chop the cucumber, leaving the skin and seeds intact.

3 Wash and roughly chop the celery leaves.

4 Place all of the ingredients into a high-speed blender and add a little more water if need be, to make up to the level of your glass.

5 Process all of the ingredients until smooth. Add a large handful of ice if desired. Enjoy immediately.

CHEF'S NOTE
Lemon verbena can offer protection against oxidative stress and has been studied at length to suggest it has great anti-oxidant properties.

MEDITERRANEAN DETOX

167 calories

Ingredients

BETA-CAROTENE →

- 150g yellow/orange bell pepper
- 250ml/8½floz coconut water
- 75g/3oz rocket leaves
- 100g/3½oz plum tomatoes
- 1 tsp rosemary leaves
- Ice cubes

Method

1 Wash and de-seed the pepper. Roughly chop.

2 Wash the rocket and rosemary leaves and drain well.

3 Wash the tomatoes and roughly chop.

4 Add all of the ingredients into a high-speed blender and top up with water if need be, to fill the glass you are using,

5 Blend until all of the ingredients are smooth. Enjoy immediately.

CHEF'S NOTE
The essential carotenoids found in peppers are essential for protection against free radicals.

GREEN LEAF CLEANSER

204 calories

Ingredients

- 125g/4oz rocket leaves
- 50g/2oz spinach leaves
- 50g/2oz butterhead lettuce
- 250ml/8½floz coconut water
- 1 tsp spirulina
- 1 tbsp pumpkin seeds
- Water

Method

1 Rinse the rocket, spinach and butterhead and drain well.

2 Add all the ingredients to a high-speed blender and add a little more water if needed, to make up to fill the glass you are using.

3 Blend until really smooth. Enjoy immediately.

CHEF'S NOTE
Spirulina is a form of blue-green algae with powerful healing and cleansing properties.

CHIA, LIME & MINT DETOX

185 calories

Ingredients

- 100g/3½oz cucumber
- 250ml/8½floz coconut water
- 1 lime
- 3 tbsp mint leaves
- 1 tbsp chia seeds
- Water

Method

1 Wash the cucumber and roughly chop, leaving the skin and seeds intact.

2 Peel the lime and roughly chop.

3 Wash and drain the mint leaves.

4 Add all of the ingredients into a high-speed blender, adding a little more water if necessary to make up to the level to fill the glass you are using.

5 Process the ingredients until smooth. You can enjoy this drink 1-2 hours after making it as the soaking chia seeds will create a thicker texture, if you prefer.

CHEF'S NOTE
Chia seeds contain high amounts of both soluble and insoluble fibre, and help to clean out the digestive tract.

CAULIFLOWER CLEANSER

162 calories

Ingredients

- 150g/5oz cauliflower
- 2 stalks of celery
- 125g/4oz white cabbage
- 250ml/8½floz coconut water
- 2 tbsp chives
- Water

Method

1 Wash the cauliflower and cut in to small florets.

2 Wash and roughly chop the celery and cabbage.

3 Wash the chives and drain well.

4 Place all of the ingredients in to a high-speed blender and add a little more water if needed, to make up to the level needed to fill the glass you are using.

5 Process the ingredients until smooth, Enjoy immediately.

CHEF'S NOTE
The glucosinolates in cauliflower activate the detoxification enzymes in our bodies.

WATERCRESS & LEMON ZINGER

194 calories

Ingredients

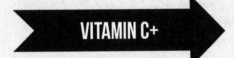
VITAMIN C+

- 250ml/8½floz coconut water
- 150g/5oz watercress
- 1 lemon
- 125g/4oz spinach
- water

Method

1 Rinse the watercress and spinach well and drain.

2 Add all the ingredients to a high-speed blender and add a little more water if need be, to make up to the level of the glass you are using.

3 Blend the ingredients until really smooth. Enjoy immediately.

CHEF'S NOTE

High in antioxidants, nutrients and vitamin C, watercress is a great detox ingredient.

ASIAN GREEN DETOX

135 calories

Ingredients

- 100g/3½oz mangetout
- 100g/3½oz bok choi
- 250ml/8½floz coconut water
- 50g/2oz bamboo shoots

- 1 pinch of chinese 5 spice
- 1 tsp grated fresh ginger

Method

1 Rinse and drain the mangetout and roughly chop.

2 Wash the bok choi and drain and split the leaves.

3 Rinse the bamboo shoots well.

4 Add all of the ingredients into a high-speed blender, adding a little water to make up to the level that will fill the glass you are using.

5 Blend the ingredients until smooth. Enjoy immediately.

CHEF'S NOTE

Bok choi is a source of quercetin, which is a powerful phytonutrient for removing free radicals from the body.

COUNTRY GARDEN CLEANSE

251 calories

- 150g/5oz Brussels sprout tops
- 50g/2oz spinach leaves
- 125g/4oz courgette
- 1 tsp sage leaves
- 1 tsp wheatgrass
- Water

Method

1 Rinse the Brussels sprout tops and spinach leaves. Roughly chop.

2 Wash and roughly chop the courgette, leaving the skin and seeds intact.

3 Wash the sage leaves and drain well.

4 Add all of the ingredients into a high-speed blender, adding a bit more water to make up the level to fill your glass.

5 Blend until smooth. Enjoy immediately.

CHEF'S NOTE
Wheatgrass is a great detox ingredient and will boost your diet with chlorophyll, to help remove toxins.

CLEANSING GOJI

172 calories

Ingredients

- 1 tbsp dried goji berries
- 1 tsp ginger root, grated
- 125g/4oz spinach leaves
- 250ml/8½floz green tea, cooled
- Water
- Ice

Method

1 Soak the goji berries in a little water for around 15 minutes.

2 Rinse and drain the spinach leaves.

3 Place all of the ingredients into a high-speed blender and top up with a little water if you want a longer drink.

4 Process the ingredients until smooth.

5 Serve with plenty of ice.

CHEF'S NOTE
Goji berries are a wonderful superfood - they're packed with antioxidants, vitamins, minerals and fibre.

KALE & FENNEL BOOST

190 calories

Ingredients

- 140g/4½oz kale
- 250ml/8½floz coconut water
- 2 stalks of celery
- 125g/4oz of cucumber

- 4-5 fennel seeds
- 1 tsp flat leaf parsley
- 1 tbsp lemon juice
- Water

Method

1 Rinse the kale well and remove any thick stalks.

2 Rinse the celery and roughly chop.

3 Clean and roughly chop the cucumber, keeping the seeds and skin intact.

4 Rinse the parsley and crush the fennel seeds a bit.

5 Add all of the ingredients into a high-speed blender, topping up with water to fill the glass you are using.

6 Blend until really smooth. Enjoy immediately.

CHEF'S NOTE
Kale is believed to help prevent cardiovascular disease, several types of cancer, asthma, rheumatoid arthritis, and premature ageing of the skin.

ROCKET BOOSTER

100 calories

Ingredients

- 250ml/8½floz coconut water
- 200g/7oz rocket leaves
- 2 tbsp lime juice

- 150g/5oz courgette
- ½ tsp oregano leaves
- water

Method

1 Rinse and drain the rocket the leaves.

2 Rinse the courgette and roughly chop, leaving the skin and seeds intact.

3 Wash the oregano leaves and drain.

4 Add all of the ingredients into a high-speed blender, topping up with water if necessary.

5 Blend the ingredients well until smooth. Enjoy immediately.

CHEF'S NOTE
Rocket leaves contain anti-oxidants that cleanse toxins and they will give you a boost of vitamin C.

Time to try....

KETO

GREEN

Smoothies

Energising

MIGHTY NUT AUBERGINE

246 calories

Ingredients

- 125g/4oz aubergine
- 1 tbsp walnuts
- 125g/4oz spinach

- 2 tbsp full fat Greek yogurt
- 100ml/3½floz coconut water
- Water

Method

1 Wash the spinach and aubergine,

2 Roughly chop the aubergine and walnuts.

3 Add the ingredients into a high-speed blender and top up with water so the level will fill the glass you are using.

4 Blend the ingredients until really smooth. Enjoy immediately.

CHEF'S NOTE
Walnuts are a great source of omega-3, the good fat that will boost energy.

SPINACH POWER

290 calories

.... *Ingredients* ....

- 150g/5oz spinach leaves
- 50g/2oz mangetout
- ½ avocado
- 4 tbsp low fat Greek yogurt

- 1 tbsp mint leaves
- 100ml/3½floz coconut water
- Water
- 2 tsp honey

.... *Method* ....

1 Rinse the spinach leaves, mint and mangetout.

2 Peel and remove the stone from the avocado.

3 Add all of the ingredients into a high-speed blender and add water if needed, so to fill the glass you will be using.

4 Blend the ingredients until really smooth. Enjoy immediately.

CHEF'S NOTE

Spinach is a good source of iron that will boost your red blood cells and the oxygen levels in your blood.

ENERGY SEED SMOOTHIE

287 calories

Ingredients

- 175ml/6floz almond milk
- 1 tbsp pumpkin seeds
- 1 tbsp chia seeds
- 75g/3oz broccoli
- 75g/3oz courgette
- 2 tbsp full fat Greek yogurt
- Water

Method

1 Rinse the broccoli and roughly chop.

2 Rinse the courgette and roughly chop, leaving the skin and seeds intact.

3 Add all the ingredients into a high-speed blender and top up with water if necessary, so it will fill the glass you are using.

4 Process the ingredients until really smooth. Enjoy immediately.

CHEF'S NOTE

Seeds are an excellent way to get some good fats and energy into a keto diet. Whilst relatively low in carbohydrates, they still pack a punch!

FLAX POWER SMOOTHIE

231 calories

.... *Ingredients* ....

- 75g/3oz radishes
- ½ avocado
- 2 tbsp flat leaf parsley

- 2 tbsp flaxseed
- 250ml/8½floz unsweetened almond milk
- Water

.... *Method* ....

1 Wash the radishes and remove the green ends.

2 Remove the stone and peel the avocado.

3 Wash and drain the parsley leaves.

4 Put all of the ingredients into a high-speed blender and add a little water if needed, so the level will fill the glass you are using.

5 Process the ingredients until smooth. Enjoy immediately.

CHEF'S NOTE

Flaxseeds are a superfood well known for their nutrients and health benefits. They are a great protein to add to a Keto diet to give you a boost in energy.

BERRY HEMP BLEND

······· *Ingredients* ·······

- ½ avocado
- 125g/4oz raspberries
- 120ml/4floz unsweetened almond milk
- 2 tbsp full fat Greek Yoghurt
- 1 tbsp hemp seeds
- Water

······· *Method* ·······

1 Rinse the raspberries.

2 Remove the peel and stone from the avocado.

3 Place all of the ingredients into a high-speed blender and add a little water if need be, so to fill the glass you are using.

4 Process the ingredients until smooth. Enjoy immediately.

CHEF'S NOTE
Berries should be used in moderation when following a Keto plan, but they can offer a welcome sweetness from time to time and they balance the flavours of the hemp seed here well,

CACAO SUPERFOOD SMOOTHIE

305 calories

Ingredients

- 250ml/8½floz coconut water
- 50g/2oz avocado
- 1 tbsp chia seeds
- 1 tbsp cacao powder
- ½ tsp vanilla extract
- 225g/8oz spinach

Method

1 Rinse the spinach well and drain.

2 Peel and de-stone the avocado.

3 Place all of the ingredients into a high-speed blender and add a little water it need be, so to make up to the level that will fill your glass.

4 Blend the ingredients until smooth. Enjoy immediately.

CHEF'S NOTE
Raw cacao contains nearly four times the antioxidant content of processed dark chocolate.

MACADAMIA & CAULIFLOWER BLAST

302 calories

Ingredients

- 225g/8oz cauliflower
- ½ avocado
- 140g/4½oz courgette
- 1 tbsp macadamia
- 250ml/8½floz unsweetened almond milk
- Water

Method

1 Rinse the cauliflower and roughly chop.

2 Rinse and roughly chop the courgette, leaving the skin and seeds intact.

3 Remove the peel and de-stone the avocado.

4 Add all of the ingredients into a high-speed blender and add a little water if necessary, so to fill the glass you are using.

5 Process the ingredients until smooth. Enjoy immediately.

CHEF'S NOTE
Macadamias are high in vitamin A, iron and protein and a tasty source of energy in a Keto diet.

RHUBARB AND GINGER SMOOTHIE

192 calories

····· *Ingredients* ·····

- 250ml/8½floz unsweetened almond milk
- ½oz avocado
- 1 tsp ginger root
- 100g/3½oz rhubarb
- 1 tsp keto sweetener of your choice
- 1 tbsp goji berries
- Water

····· *Method* ·····

1 Rinse the rhubarb and roughly chop..

2 Prepare the ginger root by grating it into a high-speed blender.

3 Add all of the ingredients to the ginger and top up with a little water if needed, so to fill the glass you are using.

4 Blend the ingredients until smooth. Enjoy immediately.

CHEF'S NOTE
Goji berries have higher levels of antioxidants than nearly all other superfoods and a great energy source.

SUPER FUEL SMOOTHIE

276 calories

Ingredients

- 200g/7oz kale
- ½ avocado
- 1 tbsp hemp seeds
- 3-4 fennel seeds
- 250ml/8½floz unsweetened almond milk
- Water
- Ice

Method

1 Rinse the kale and remove any thick stems.

2 Peel the avocado and remove the stone.

3 Crush the fennel seeds a little.

4 Add all of the ingredients into a high-speed blender and add a little water if need be, so the level will fill the glass you are using,

5 Blend until smooth. Enjoy immediately with plenty of ice.

CHEF'S NOTE
Make sure you use unsweetened almond milk when making Keto smoothies.

WATERCRESS CREAM SMOOTHIE

170 calories

Ingredients

- 225g/8oz watercress
- 75g/3oz cucumber
- 2 tbsp single cream
- 250ml/8½floz unsweetened almond milk
- 1 tbsp ground almonds
- Water

Method

1 Rinse the watercress and drain well.

2 Rinse and roughly chop the cucumber, leaving the skin and seeds intact.

3 Add all of the ingredients into a high-speed blender and add a little water so the level will fill the glass you are using.

4 Process the ingredients until smooth. Enjoy immediately.

CHEF'S NOTE
The added ground almonds create more creaminess and brings energy and fibre to this smoothie.

SPICE ENERGISER

162 calories

.... *Ingredients* ....

- 120ml/4floz coconut water
- 175g/6oz aubergine
- 1 orange or red bell pepper
- 1 tsp turmeric

- 1/2 tsp cumin
- 1 tbsp cashew nuts
- water

.... *Method* ....

1 Wash the aubergine and roughly chop.

2 Wash and remove the seeds from the pepper and roughly chop.

3 Roughly chop the cashews.

4 Add all of the ingredients into a high-speed blender and add a little water if needed so the level will fill the glass you are using.

5 Blend the ingredients until smooth. Enjoy immediately.

CHEF'S NOTE
Try soaking the cashew nuts in water overnight to create an even creamier drink.

COCONUT SPINACH SMOOTHIE

375 calories

Ingredients

- 225g/8oz spinach
- 2 tbsp coconut cream
- ½ avocado
- 1 tbsp hemp seeds
- 200ml/7floz coconut water
- Water

Method

1 Rinse the spinach well and drain.

2 Remove the skin and stone from the avocado.

3 Add all of the ingredients into a high-speed blender and add a little water if necessary so it comes to a level that will fill the glass you are using.

4 Process the ingredients until smooth. Enjoy immediately.

CHEF'S NOTE
Make sure you use the full fat version of coconut mik to get the best energy hit.

EXOTIC SUMAC BOOST

279 calories

Ingredients

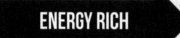

ENERGY RICH

- 200g/7oz cauliflower
- 1 tsp sumac
- 1 tbsp flaxseed
- 250ml/8 ½floz unsweetened almond milk
- 100g/3½oz avocado
- Water

Method

1 Rinse the cauliflower and cut into florets.

2 Peel and stone the avocado.

3 Add all of the ingredients into a high-speed blender and add a little water if need be, to make up to the level to fill the glass you are using.

4 Process the ingredients until smooth. Enjoy immediately.

CHEF'S NOTE
Sumac is a widely used spice, tasting of mild peppery, lemon. It is considered a great anti-inflammatory ingredient.

GREEN TEA COOL FUEL

188 calories

Ingredients

- 250ml/8½floz green tea, cooled
- ½ avocado
- 3 tbsp full fat Greek yoghurt
- 200g/7oz cucumber
- 1 tsp matcha powder
- 2 tsp mint leaves
- Water

Method

1 Wash and roughly chop the cucumber, leaving the seeds and skin intact.

2 Rinse and drain the mint leaves.

3 Add all of the ingredients into a high-speed blender and add a little more water if you want a longer drink.

4 Process the ingredients until everything is really smooth. Serve immediately.

CHEF'S NOTE
Matcha powder is full of vitamin C, selenium, zinc and magnesium.

FUEL STOP SMOOTHIE

340 calories

Ingredients

COMFORTING ENERGY

- ½ avocado
- 1 tsp vanilla extract
- 2 tbsp macadamia
- 2 tbsp full fat Greek yoghurt
- 200ml/7floz coconut milk
- water

Method

1 Peel and stone the avocado.

2 Chop the macadamia nuts a little to help with blending.

3 Add all of the ingredients into a high-speed blender and add a little water if needed, so the level will fill the glass you are using.

4 Process the ingredients until smooth.

5 Enjoy immediately.

CHEF'S NOTE
This smoothie is full of good fats and low carbohydrates. It's an excellent choice for when you feel you need a hit of energy but don't fancy lots of green veg!

SPICED GREEN SMOOTHIE

Ingredients

- 75g/3oz kale
- 2 celery stalks
- ½ tsp spirulina
- 1 pinch ground cinnamon
- 1 tsp grated ginger root
- 175ml/6oz unsweetened almond milk
- 3 tbsp full fat Greek Yoghurt
- Water

Method

1 Rinse the kale and the celery. Chop the celery and remove the thick stems from the kale.

2 Add all the ingredients to a high-speed blender. Top with a little water so the level will the glass you are using,

3 Process the ingredients until smooth. Enjoy immediately.

CHEF'S NOTE
Spirulina is a great source of nutrients including vitamins B, C, D, A and E and worth stocking for Keto plans.

HEMP & SWEET PEPPER SMOOTHIE

320 calories

Ingredients

- 225g/8oz spinach
- 60g/2oz yellow or orange pepper
- 1 stalk celery
- 1 tbsp hemp seeds
- ½ avocado

- 175ml/6oz unsweetened almond milk
- 2 tbsp full fat Greek Yoghurt
- ½ tsp oregano leaves
- Water

Method

1 Rinse the spinach, oregano, pepper and celery.

2 De-seed the pepper. Peel & de-stone the avocado.

3 Rinse and roughly chop the celery.

4 Add all of the ingredients to a high-speed blender and top up with water if necessary so the level will fill the glass you are using,

5 Process until smooth. Enjoy immediately.

CHEF'S NOTE
Make sure you use full fat Greek yoghurts when preparing keto smoothies,

CUCUMBER & DILL NUTTER

254 calories

Ingredients

- 5 sprigs fresh dill
- 300g/11oz cucumber
- 250ml/8½floz unsweetened almond milk
- ½ avocado
- 10 raw pistachio nuts
- Water
- Ice cubes

Method

1 Roughly chop the cucumber, leaving the skin and seeds intact.

2 Wash the dill and drain well.

3 Peel & de-stone the avocado.

4 Add all of the ingredients to a high speed blender and top up with a little water if need be, so to fill the glass you will be using.

5 Blend the ingredients until really smooth. Enjoy immediately.

CHEF'S NOTE
Pistachios are a good source of fibre, protein, and heart-healthy fats.

VEG HEAD

309 calories

Ingredients

- 250ml/8½floz unsweetened almond milk
- 225g/8oz spinach
- 175g/6oz tomatoes
- 150g/5oz courgette
- ½ avocado
- 1 tbsp hemp seeds
- water

Method

1 Rinse the spinach, tomatoes & courgettes and roughly chop.

2 Peel and de-stone the avocado.

3 Add all of the ingredients to a high-speed blender, topping up with water if needed, so you can fill the glass you are using,

4 Process the ingredients until really smooth. Enjoy immediately.

CHEF'S NOTE

Blender Tip....if you sometimes find your ingredients won't all fit in your cup under the max line. Try blending some together first to make room for the other ingredients.

VEGGIE HAZELNUT SMOOTHIE

392 calories

Ingredients

- ½ avocado
- 150g/5oz cucumber
- 1 tbsp hazelnuts
- 125g/4oz tomatoes
- 75g/3oz kale
- 1 tbsp lemon juice
- 250ml/8½floz unsweetened almond milk
- Water

Method

1 Rinse the kale and remove any tough stems.

2 Peel and de-stone the avocado.

3 Wash and roughly chop the cucumber, keeping the skin and seeds intact.

4 Wash the tomatoes and roughly chop.

5 Add all of the ingredients to a high-speed blender, topping up with a little water if you need to so you can fill the glass you will be using.

6 Blend the ingredients together until really smooth. Enjoy immediately.

CHEF'S NOTE
Hazelnuts are a rich source of dietary fibre, manganese, vitamin B1, and the essential fatty acid omega-3.

DOUBLE ALMOND BOOST

389 calories

Ingredients

- 75g/3oz cucumber
- 50g/2oz avocado
- 1 tbsp almond butter
- 2cm/1inch piece fresh root ginger
- 1 tsp ground cinnamon
- 225g/8oz spinach
- 200ml/7floz unsweetened almond milk
- Water

Method

1 Rinse the spinach & cucumber and roughly chop.

2 Peel and de-stone the avocado.

3 Peel and grate the ginger.

4 Add all the ingredients to a high-speed blender and top with a little water if needed, so you can fill the glass you are going to use.

5 Blend the ingredients until smooth. Enjoy immediately.

CHEF'S NOTE
Almond butter is a source of vitamin E, copper, magnesium, and high quality protein.

RED DEVIL BOOST

288 calories

Ingredients

- 200g/7oz tomato
- 60g/2oz red pepper
- 75g/3oz romaine lettuce
- ½ avocado
- ½ tsp ground cinnamon
- Pinch of cayenne pepper
- 1 tbsp Brazil nuts
- 200ml/7oz coconut water
- Water

Method

1 Rinse the tomato, pepper and lettuce. Core and roughly chop the pepper.

2 Peel and de-stone the avocado.

3 Chop the Brazil nuts a little to help blending.

4 Add all of the ingredients to a high-speed blender and top up with water if need be, so the level will fill the glass you are using.

5 Process the ingredients until smooth. Enjoy immediately.

CHEF'S NOTE
Tomatoes are an excellent source of vitamin C and add a natural sweetness to keto dishes.

GET UP THYME

215 calories

Ingredients

- 150g/5oz cucumber
- 1 tbsp fresh thyme
- 225g/8oz spinach
- 1 tbsp lemon juice
- ½ avocado
- 1 tbsp ground almonds
- 250ml/8½floz coconut water
- Water

Method

1 Rinse the cucumber, thyme and spinach.

2 Roughly chop the cucumber, keeping the skin and seeds intact..

3 Peel and de-stone the avocado.

4 Add all of the ingredients to a high-speed blender and top with a little water if needed, so it will fill the glass you are using.

5 Blend the ingredients until smooth. Enjoy immediately.

CHEF'S NOTE
Thyme is rich in many vital vitamins, including Vitamin C, B 12, K and A.

MEAN GREEN MACHINE

273 calories

Ingredients

- 50g/2oz broccoli
- 75g/3oz kale
- 225g/8oz spinach
- ½ avocado
- 1 tbsp lemon juice

- 1 tsp chia seeds
- 1 tsp matcha powder
- 200ml/7floz coconut water
- Water

Method

1 Wash the broccoli, kale and spinach. Cut any thick stems off the kale.

2 Peel and de-stone the avocado.

3 Put all of the ingredients into a high-speed blender and add a little water if needed, so to fill the glass you are using.

4 Process the ingredients until smooth. Enjoy immediately.

CHEF'S NOTE
This smoothie contains a huge spectrum of vitamins and minerals and is a good meal replacement.

ENDIVE ENERGY

348 calories

······· *Ingredients* ·······

- ½ avocado
- 150g/5oz endive
- 225g/8oz spinach
- 1 celery stalk

- 250ml/8½floz unsweetened almond milk
- 1 tbsp flat leaf parsley
- Water

······· *Method* ·······

1 Wash the endive, parsley and spinach and drain well.

2 Peel and de-stone the avocado.

3 Add all of the ingredients to a high-speed blender and add a little water if needed, to make up to the level that will fill the glass you are using.

4 Process the ingredients until smooth. Enjoy immediately.

CHEF'S NOTE
Almond milk is high in energy, proteins, lipids and fibre.

CASHEW BUTTER & SPINACH SMOOTHIE

396 calories

Ingredients

- 1 tbsp cashew butter
- 1 tbsp cashews
- 225g/8oz spinach
- 100g/3½oz avocado
- 250ml coconut water
- Ice cubes

Method

1 Rinse the spinach well and drain.

2 Peel and de-stone the avocado.

3 Add all the ingredients to a high-speed blender and add a little water if need be, so to fill the glass you are using.

4 Blend the ingredients until smooth. Enjoy immediately.

CHEF'S NOTE
Vary the nuts and nut butter to suit your own taste, they will all provide you with a great boost of energy.

DECONSTRUCTED PESTO SMOOTHIE

266 calories

Ingredients

CALCIUM HIT

- 150g/5oz rocket leaves
- ½ avocado
- 1 tbsp pine nuts
- 250ml/8½floz unsweetened almond milk
- 1 garlic clove
- 1 tbsp parmesan cheese
- Water

Method

1 Wash the rocket and drain well.

2 Crush the pine nuts a little and crush the garlic clove.

3 Add all of the ingredients to a high-speed blender and top up with a little water if need be, so it will fill the glass you are using.

4 Process the ingredients until smooth. Enjoy immediately.

CHEF'S NOTE

This is a great smoothie if you need a calcium boost, your bones and teeth will thank you for it!

PUMPKIN SEED RUSH

421 calories

Ingredients

- ½ avocado
- 2 tbsp pumpkin seeds
- 125g/4oz kale
- 125g/4oz cucumber
- 250ml/8½floz unsweetened almond milk
- Water

Method

1 Peel and remove the stone in the avocado.

2 Wash and drain the kale, removing any thick stems.

3 Rinse and roughly chop the cucumber, keeping the skin and seeds intact.

4 Add all of the ingredients to a high-speed blender and add a little water if need be, so the level will fill the glass you are using.

5 Process the ingredients until smooth. Enjoy immediately.

CHEF'S NOTE
You could also use other milk as an alternative, but choose ones that are low in sugar and carbohydrates..

HERB BULLET

358 calories

Ingredients

- ½ avocado
- 225g/8oz spinach
- 2 tbsp walnuts
- 200ml/7floz bone broth

- 1 tbsp flat leaf parsley
- 1 tbsp chives
- 1 tbsp thyme leaves
- 1 tsp coconut oil

Method

1 Rinse the spinach and drain.

2 Rinse and drain the herbs.

3 Add all of the ingredients to a high-speed blender.

4 Blend until everything is smooth.

5 Enjoy immediately.

CHEF'S NOTE
This savoury smoothie is full of flavour and a great hit of nutrition for a keto plan.

SUPER GREEN SHOT

245 calories

Ingredients

- 1 tsp spirulina
- 1 tbsp hemp seed
- 125g/4oz broccoli
- 125g/4oz kale
- 125g/green cabbage
- 120ml/4floz bone broth

Method

1 Wash and roughly cut the cabbage, kale and broccoli, removing any tough stems or stalks.

2 Add everything to a high-speed blender. This is a really short drink, so don't add any extra water. You could even serve in shot glasses.

3 Blend the ingredients until really smooth. Enjoy immediately.

CHEF'S NOTE
Bone broth has great healing properties and a wealth of protein building blocks.

NUTTY LEMON LIFT

288 calories

Ingredients

- 1 tbsp brazil nuts
- 200g/7oz courgette
- 2 tbsp full fat Greek Yoghurt
- 200ml/7floz unsweetened almond milk
- 1 tsp lemon verbena leaves
- 1 lemon
- Pinch ground cardamom
- Water

Method

1 Wash and roughly chop the courgette, leaving the skin and seeds intact.

2 Wash and drain the lemon verbena leaves.

3 Roughly chop the brazil nuts, to help the blending.

4 Add all of the ingredients to a high-speed blender and add a little more water if need be so the level will fill the glass you are using.

5 Process until smooth and enjoy immediately.

CHEF'S NOTE

Brazil nuts are a source of selenium and will give both your mood and your energy a lift.

RHUBARB & CUSTARD ENERGISER

304 calories

Ingredients

- 100g/3½oz rhubarb
- ½ avocado
- 200ml/7floz unsweetened almond milk
- 2 tbsp pecan nuts
- ½ tsp nutmeg
- 1 tsp vanilla extract
- 2 tbsp single cream
- Water

Method

1 Wash and roughly chop the rhubarb.

2 Remove the peel and de-stone the avocado.

3 Roughly chop the pecans a little.

4 Add all of the ingredients to a high-speed blender and top up with water if need be, to enable you to fill the glass you are using.

5 Blend the ingredients well, until really smooth. Enjoy immediately.

CHEF'S NOTE
These flavours are similar to this classic combo and the added pecans provide protein to help energise you.

FLAX FUSE

286 calories

Ingredients

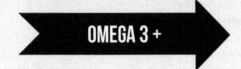
OMEGA 3 +

- 2 tbsp flaxseeds
- ½ avocado
- 125g/4oz cucumber
- 200ml/7floz coconut water
- Water
- Ice cubes

Method

1 Remove the peel and de-stone the avocado.

2 Wash and roughly chop the cucumber, keeping the skin and seeds intact.

3 Add all of the ingredients to a high-speed blender, adding water if need be to the level that will fill the glass you are using.

4 Process the ingredients until really smooth. Enjoy immediately with ice for an extra cold drink.

CHEF'S NOTE
Flaxseeds are a source of energy and lignans, compounds thought to reduce risk of developing certain cancers.

BUTTER BOOST SMOOTHIE

189 calories

Ingredients

FIBRE PROVIDER

- 150g/5oz frozen blueberries
- 1 tbsp almond butter
- 1 tbsp tahini
- 300ml/10½ floz coconut water
- Ice

Method

1 Don't defrost the blueberries - use them straight from the freezer.

2 Add all of the ingredients to a high-speed blender, except the ice.

3 Blend the ingredients until smooth.

4 Top with a large handful of ice and enjoy this slushie smoothie immediately.

CHEF'S NOTE
Berries can be used in a Keto plan and they are full of health boosting flavanoids, but only consume in moderation.

GINGER PUNCH

339 calories

Ingredients

- 200g/7oz cucumber
- 2 tsp ginger root, grated
- ½ avocado
- 1 tbsp macadamia nuts
- 200ml/7floz hemp milk
- Water

Method

1 Wash and roughly chop the cucumber, keeping the skin and seeds intact.

2 Remove the peel and de-stone the avocado.

3 Prepare the ginger and add to a high-speed blender.

4 Add all of the other ingredients to the blender and top with a little water if needed, to make the level up to be able to fill your glass.

5 Process the ingredients until smooth. Enjoy immediately.

CHEF'S NOTE
Ginger is known for it's wonderful anti-inflammatory properties and is a great addition to a keto diet.

NUTTY GREEN BOOST

406 calories

Ingredients

- 225g/8oz spinach
- ½ avocado
- 1 tbsp chopped fresh lemon verbena

- 2tbsp almond butter
- 200ml/7floz unsweetened almond milk
- Water

Method

1 Rinse the spinach.

2 Peel and de-stone the avocado.

3 Rinse and dry the lemon verbena leaves.

4 Add all of the ingredients into a high-speed blender and top up with a little water if need be so it will fill the glass you are using.

5 Process the ingredients until smooth. Enjoy immediately.

CHEF'S NOTE
Almonds are a great source of protein and magnesium and will help keep you feeling fuller for longer.

Time to try....

KETO

GREEN

SMOOTHIES

Full Keto

BULLETPROOF COFFEE SMOOTHIE

402 calories

Ingredients

ENERGY TREAT

- 250ml/8½floz coffee
- 1 tbsp coconut oil, melted
- 1 tbsp butter, melted
- 1 tsp vanilla extract
- 1/2 tsp cinnamon
- 4 tbsp whipping cream
- ice to serve

Method

1 Place all of the ingredients, apart from the ice, into a high-speed blender.

2 Blend the ingredients until the whipping cream starts to thicken and froth.

3 Pour into a glass and top with plenty of ice.

CHEF'S NOTE
Bulletproof coffee is a Keto friendly energy boosting drink and this iced smoothie version is a great start to a summer's morning.

CHOCOMINT SMOOTHIE

145 calories

······· *Ingredients* ·······

FLAVANOIDS +

- 1 tbsp single cream
- 1 tbsp raw cacao powder
- 2 tbsp mint leaves
- 250m/8½floz coconut water
- Water

······· *Method* ·······

1 Wash and drain the mint leaves (you could use any variety of mint leaves for this recipe; the chocolate mint leaf goes really well).

2 Place the cream, cacao powder, mint and coconut water into a high-speed blender.

3 Process the ingredients until all of the ingredients are really smooth.

4 Serve in a glass with an extra sprinkle of cacao powder and an optional spoonful of thick, whipped cream.

CHEF'S NOTE
Try with any unsweetened Keto friendly milk for this recipe.

PROTEIN BERRY BLAST

209 calories

Ingredients

BOOSTS ENERGY

- 175g/6oz strawberries
- 1 tbsp hemp seed
- 1 tbsp sunflower seeds
- 250ml/8½ floz unsweetened almond milk
- Water

Method

1 Rinse and hull the strawberries. Roughly chop.

2 Add all of the ingredients to a high-speed blender and top with a little water if need be, so you can fill the glass you are using.

3 Blend the ingredients until smooth. Serve immediately.

CHEF'S NOTE

Protein is vital to muscle growth and tissue repair and is found in hemp and sunflower seeds.

STRAWBERRIES & CREAM

259 calories

····· *Ingredients* ·····

- 175g/6oz strawberries
- 3 tbsp single cream
- 200ml/7floz unsweetened almond milk

- 1 tsp vanilla extract
- A few mint leaves to serve
- Ice to serve

····· *Method* ·····

1 Rinse and hull the strawberries and roughly chop.

2 Place all of the ingredients into a high-speed blender and top up with water if need be, so you can fill the glass you are using.

3 Blend the ingredients until really smooth.

4 Enjoy immediately with mint leaves and plenty of ice.

CHEF'S NOTE
Strawberries can be eaten in moderation when you have balanced your Keto diet, just be sure to not over do them!

MIDDLE EASTERN PROMISE

387 calories

Ingredients

FIBRE RICH →

- 200g/7oz blackberries
- 50g/2oz blueberries
- 1 tbsp brazil nuts
- 100ml/3½oz full fat Greek yogurt
- 200ml/7floz almond milk
- Water

Method

1 Rinse and drain the blackberries and blueberries,

2 Add all of the ingredients to a high-speed blender and top up with a little water if needed, so the level will fill the glass you are using.

3 Blend the ingredients until smooth. Enjoy immediately.

CHEF'S NOTE
Blackberries are a great source of manganese.

ALMOND & CHIA SMOOTHIE

317 calories

Ingredients

- ½ avocado
- 2 tbsp almond butter
- 250ml/ 8½floz unsweetened almond milk
- 1 tbsp chia seeds
- Water

Method

1 Remove the peel and de-stone the avocado.

2 Place the avocado flesh, almond butter, almond milk and chia seeds into a high speed blender, adding a little more water if necessary so you can fill the glass you are using.

3 Process the ingredients until really smooth.

4 Serve immediately.

CHEF'S NOTE
Almonds can add magnesium to your diet, which promotes blood flow to the heart.

COCONUT BERRY BLAST

238 calories

Ingredients

CLEANSING

- 150g/5oz mixed berries (blueberries, raspberries or blackberries)
- 250ml/8½floz coconut water
- 1 tbsp coconut cream
- 15g/½oz pumpkin seeds
- Water

Method

1 Wash and drain the berries.

2 Add the coconut water, coconut cream and pumpkin seeds to a high-speed blender and top up with water if needed, so you can fill the glass you are using.

3 Blend the ingredients until they are smooth.

4 Serve immediately.

CHEF'S NOTE
Use the thick coconut cream block here to add with the milk as it will bring a lovely depth of coconut flavour to this drink.

COFFEE & CINNAMON BOOST

126 calories

Ingredients

- ½ tsp cinnamon
- 3 tbsp single cream
- 200ml/7floz coffee, cooled
- ½ tsp vanilla
- Ice

Method

1 Add all of the ingredients into a high-speed blender and add a handful of ice.

2 Process until the ingredients are well mixed and the ice has broken down.

3 Serve this iced smoothie immediately.

CHEF'S NOTE

Experiment with more cinnamon and even some nutmeg too, for a warmer, spicier taste.

RASPBERRY & WHITE CHOCOLATE COOLER

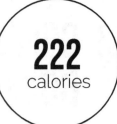

222 calories

Ingredients

GOOD FATS

- 200g/7oz raspberries
- 1 tsp cocoa butter
- ½ tsp coconut oil, melted
- 200ml/7floz unsweetened almond milk
- 1 tsp vanilla extract
- Ice

Method

1 Rinse the raspberries well.

2 Add all of the ingredients to a high-speed blender. apart from the ice.

3 Blend the ingredients until smooth.

4 Add a handful of ice to the cooler and serve immediately,

CHEF'S NOTE
Try and find raw cocoa butter as it has a higher level of nutrients.

GINGERBREAD FAT BOMB SMOOTHIE

220
calories

Ingredients

- 1 tsp ground ginger
- 1 tsp ground cinnamon
- 1 tbsp almond flour
- 1 tbsp almond butter

- ½ tsp stevia/Keto sweetener
- 200ml/7oz coconut milk
- 2 tbsp melted butter
- 1 tbsp lemon juice

Method

1 Put all of the ingredients into a high-speed blender.

2 Process until everything is well combined and smooth.

3 Add a little more stevia/sweetener to taste and serve immediately.

CHEF'S NOTE

This high energy and high fat smoothie is perfect for those following a Keto diet.

LEMON CHEESECAKE SMOOTHIE

182 calories

Ingredients

CALCIUM BOOST

- 1 lemon, zest and juice
- 4 tbsp cream cheese
- 200ml/7floz unsweetened almond milk
- ½ tsp ground ginger
- Water

Method

1 Wash the lemon and zest it. Squeeze all of the juice out (try rolling this on the worktop with a firm hand beforehand so the juice is easier to squeeze).

2 Add all of the ingredients to a high-speed blender, topping up with a little water if needed, so you can fill the glass you are using.

3 Blend the ingredients until smooth.

4 Enjoy immediately.

CHEF'S NOTE
Lemons are full of vitamin C and a great anti-oxidant.

GOOSEBERRY BOMB

345 calories

Ingredients

- 175g/6oz gooseberries
- ½ avocado
- 1 tbsp mint leaves
- 1 tbsp chia seeds

- 2 tbsp single cream
- 250ml/8 floz unsweetened almond milk
- 1 tbsp chia seeds
- Water

Method

1 Rinse and drain the gooseberries, removing any stalks.

2 Peel and de-stone the avocado.

3 Add all of the ingredients to a high-speed blender, topping up with a little water if need be, so you can fill the glass you are using.

4 Blend until all of the ingredients are blended. Enjoy immediately.

CHEF'S NOTE
Gooseberries are a good source of vitamin C, manganese and dietary fibre.

RASPBERRY SALAD SHAKE

288 calories

Ingredients

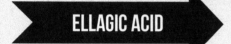

ELLAGIC ACID

- 200g/7floz raspberries
- 125g/4oz rocket leaves
- ½ avocado
- 1 tsp oregano leaves
- 200ml/7floz unsweetened almond milk
- Water

Method

1 Rinse the raspberries and drain.

2 Peel and de-stone the avocado.

3 Wash and drain the rocket and oregano.

4 Add all of the ingredients to a high-speed blender and add a little water if need be, so the level will fill the glass you are using.

5 Blend until smooth. Enjoy immediately.

CHEF'S NOTE
The ellagic acid in raspberries is thought to be a useful compound in reducing the risk of developing some cancers.